MW00961657

Living Well

A series of short articles for holistic living

by Surina Ann Jordan

Zima Health Publishing Division
P.O. Box 65204
Baltimore, MD 21209

www.zimahealth.com

Fourth Edition

Table of Contents

"This little book was developed in hopes that the spirit within you will use this information to remind you of what you already know, and show you the path to live it!"

—Surina Ann Jordan

3

Healthy Eating: An Investment in Your Future

Quality of life comes from an investment in a healthy lifestyle. Old age and poor health do not come bundled together in some inevitable fate. We can intervene. Better yet, we can prevent many of the illnesses we typically face.

If you envision what you would like to do and how you would choose to live 10 or 20 years from now, it is all possible if you maintain your health, strength, and a sound mind. In order to get there, you must define the path and the plan that will help you achieve that goal, and then pursue it aggressively and with excitement!

Food is power!

You do not have to wait until the plan fully matures; often these types of investments yield immediate benefits. If you currently drink little water, an increase of just two or three glasses each day will yield better elimination of waste and clearer skin within days! Walking one mile three times a week improves digestion, redistributes body weight, improves posture, and helps you sleep better!

In 24 months, every cell in your body is replaced. What you eat and how you care for yourself affects the quality of your new cells. Eating more raw fruits, vegetables, and whole grains and less fried and processed food will help provide resources the body needs to build good cells and protect your future health.

Poor health is a high-risk proposition based on decisions that we make every day. Sickness and disease rob us of our independence and quality of life. It is a good idea to hedge yourself against the rapid decline of good health by developing a healthy lifestyle as an investment strategy for your future.

Developing Your Baseline for Health

It is essential to get certain exams and tests each year to develop a baseline of information about your state of health. A baseline indicates what condition you are in at a given point in time. This is important so that if a symptom or health problem should arise, you have a sense of when the problem started or from where it originated.

Your health baseline should include a set of annual check-ups and exams, such as:	
Women	• Pelvic exam (pap test) • Professional breast exam • Bone density test • Tests for diseases/disorders in your family history (i.e. cancer, stroke, reproductive issues)
Men	• Digital rectal exam • PSA (Prostate-Specific Antigen) test • Tests for diseases/disorders in your family history (i.e. heart disease, high blood pressure)

There are many alternative, preventive measures that strengthen the immune system when added to your baseline regimen. For example, a full body massage improves circulation and decreases stress, while chiropractic adjustments help maintain spinal health and hip alignment.

Studies show that many ailments can be triggered by stress or other emotional trauma, such as the death of a loved one, loss of employment, divorce, or injury. Major changes that disrupt your life can cause the immune system to be compromised and make you vulnerable to sickness and disease.

Studies show that many ailments can be triggered by stress.

With an up-to-date health baseline, it is easier to determine the root causes of changes in your health.

Weight Loss – The Bigger Issue

Today, we are all in a battle against the popular culture and daily pressures that make it far too convenient to be overweight. Without thinking, we eat and live out what is presented to us. Social events, peer and family pressure, and constant advertisements all scream "Eat! Eat as much as you want!" According to the annual State of Obesity: Better Policies for a Healthier America, more than 30 percent of adults, nearly 17 percent of children ages two to 19, were found to be obese.

It is very easy to accept being overweight. No matter what weight we are, we can find beautiful clothes, and there will always be someone who is "fatter than me." We will always know someone who is being medicated for high blood pressure, diabetes, allergies, or worse. Excess body weight is a major risk factor in all of these conditions.

"The body is a mirror that reflects the food we eat."

—Unknown

Weight gain is gradual. To stay a healthy weight, avoid crash diets and instead make permanent changes that benefit your health. Eat more fresh fruit and vegetables. Eliminate fried and fast food. Exercise and drink water. Carry your own healthy snacks with you to avoid the temptation to buy something unhealthy when you are hungry.

Watch your portions. Get the maximum nutritional value from every calorie. The food industry produces about 3800 calories a day for every person in the United States. The average woman requires 2200 per day.[*] Men require about 2400 calories per day. To calculate the number of calories required for your body weight, multiply your weight times 10, then increase that number by 30 percent. All excess calories will be converted to fat. Reduce weight by reducing calories. Don't expect rapid weight loss; two to four pounds per week is the average rate of weight loss.

Average Calories Per Day for Maintaining Current Weight	
Women (age 19-50)	• 2200-2400 calories (active lifestyle) • 2000-2200 calories (moderate lifestyle) • 1800-2000 calories (sedentary lifestyle)
Men (age 19-50)	• 2800-3000 calories (active lifestyle) • 2400-2800 calories (moderate lifestyle) • 2200-2600 calories (sedentary lifestyle)

Combating and preventing weight gain and other chronic diseases also requires spiritual awakening of self, as it relates to one's divine purpose. It requires going deep into that uncharted territory to understand, "What legacy or difference will I make on earth before I leave?" You then realize that it's not about weight loss at all! It is about you caring enough to make changes and develop a healthy, planned lifestyle that allows you to accomplish your purpose-driven responsibilities.

---

[*] Reference:
USDA's Center for Nutrition Policy and Promotion; USDA's Economic Research Service.

Foundations for Living Naturally

With the abundance of chocolate, caffeine, alcohol, antidepressants, video games, cell phones, television, and the Internet, we can easily cope with the pressures of life. We no longer have to think deeply, reflect, plan, or work for change. Life can go on.

Stress, poor health, and a sense of lack has made many of us feel like prisoners. We have lost our enthusiasm for life and all it has to offer. We have lost real consciousness for living and, as a result, we have deferred our dreams and aspirations. Discouragement of our ideas has helped settle that. Now, we are full throttle in "survival mode" and seemingly content living this way.

Deep on the inside, however, is a little eternal flame that burns within the spirit—a flame that is the center of wholeness and well-being. The spirit is the central intelligence that connects us to the Creator of the universe. That intelligence has no boundaries, makes order within chaos, and maintains a rhythm to which everything living responds.

> Deep on the inside is a flame that is the center of wholeness and well-being.

Catherine Ponder, author of *The Dynamic Laws of Healing* (California: DeVorss & Company, 1966), states, "Choosing life without the spirit of the Creator is the root of all sickness and disease." Someone once said that sickness and disease is symptomatic of a poor spirit, a broken heart, and a confused mind.

Gary Gunderson, former director of the Interfaith Health Program at the Rollins School of Public Health at Emory University, states in his book *Boundary Leaders* (Fortress Press, 2004) that "if there are not resolutions to issues, then the body will find a way to die." Issues (mind, body, or spirit) created by dysfunctional or abusive lifestyles threaten the state of health and take us further away from the path of natural living.

To live naturally we must stay with the rhythm of the Creator and add fuel to that little flame inside by acknowledging its presence and value in our lives. The foundations of natural living are gifts from the Creator. These foundations include clean air and water, sunshine, rain, rich soil, vegetation, and peace.

In our current digital age, sticking to the basics is often a challenge. We need to manage technology and not let technology manage us. It is important to do all things in moderation. We need chemical-free food, water, rest, exercise, positive thoughts and relationships, self-acceptance, and meaningful livelihoods.

> We need to manage technology and not let technology manage us.

If we can stick to the basics, we can lead from within. The power, peace, and purpose within us will be given a chance to heal us. And just as important, we will be able to heal the world around us in ways we previously never imagined. This is the foundation for living naturally!

Refined Sugar: The Sweet Enemy

Refined white sugar is in almost everything we eat. It is in the loaf of bread we buy, that great jar of pasta sauce, and even in peanut butter! One can of regular soda has 12 teaspoons of sugar. Not only is sugar overused, it's used more widespread than most of us realize.

One can of regular soda has 12 teaspoons of sugar.

"What's wrong with this?" you might ask. Refined sugar impacts blood sugar levels, which can lead to diabetes, high cholesterol, and weight gain.[*] The average American consumes 30 pounds of sugar every year. Some question if it should be called a food or a drug. It is rapidly absorbed into the bloodstream. Over time, it may permanently affect the body's ability to regulate blood sugar levels, causing low blood sugar or diabetes. It is also linked to weight increase, loss of appetite, decreased libido, fatigue, tooth decay, depression, and rheumatism. Difficulty thinking and increased hyperactivity can also be added to this list.

Refined sugar can cause fatigue, depression, difficulty concentrating, hypertension, and even decreased libido.

Refined sugar has been stripped of all nutrients during the refinement and bleaching processes. The absence of these nutrients makes it an incomplete food that cannot be metabolized. When eaten, a "sugar rush" occurs, which many mistake as a source of energy. In reality, it is the body in crisis. The stomach is paralyzed until acids are mobilized to neutralize it. The production of acids is counteracted by an emergency mobilization of stored minerals. In other words, the body begins to take nutrients (mainly minerals) from itself. These minerals are pulled from different areas of the body, like the heart, kidneys, liver, and nervous system causing deficiencies and complications, including mood swings.

Natural sugar has less impact than refined sugar does on the balance of high and low blood sugar levels.

Natural sugar obtained from fruits, grains, and vegetables is absorbed into the bloodstream gradually and has less impact on the balance of high and low blood sugar levels. Other natural sweeteners include molasses, maple syrup, agave nectar, fruit juice, barley malt, raw honey, raisins, and dates. Natural sugar contains the vitamins and minerals the body needs to metabolize sugar without crisis.

Natural sugar, like any food, should be used in moderation.

------

[*] Reference:
WebMD. "The Truth about Sugar." http://www.webmd.com/food-recipes/features/health-effects-of-sugar.

Staying Young and Well with Food

The typical American diet is a blessing and a curse. It is a blessing that we have access to a large variety of foods that are reasonably priced, easy to prepare, and taste good. It is a curse, however, for almost the same reasons. Convenience makes it easy to choose foods we like, not necessarily those the body needs. Many of the most convenient foods do not provide the nutritional components the body needs to maintain good health.

A proper, plant-based diet keeps the body clean and functioning well. Foods that have lots of fiber and water, and little to no refined sugar or saturated fat, help the body. High fiber foods include whole-grain breads, cereals, rice, beans, and pasta. High water foods include fresh (and frozen) vegetables and fruits of all types. Three or four servings per day is ideal.

Fruits and vegetables scrub the inside of the body.

Fresh vegetables and fruits contain chlorophyll and other nutrients that support immune function. Five to six servings per day of these foods is best. A serving is generally a 1/2 cup, or a baseball size piece of fruit. The body uses these foods to scrub and loosen residue, which helps maintain health. The secret to youthful skin and more energy is to expel waste out of the body as soon as possible. This prevents excessive cell damage, age lines, and joint pain.

You do not have to become a vegetarian in order to look young and healthy. However, a conscious effort must be made to provide the body with the foods it needs to stay healthy. Avoid eating excessive meat and fried foods. Let meat (or fish) be a side dish.

> You do not have to become a vegetarian in order to look young and healthy.

A diet based on plants protects against early aging and many diseases that are extremely common. The right food choices can help keep us young and well!

Eating Quality Food for Colon Health

There is a body of evidence that suggests the microbial community within the intestines impacts the body's immune system.* Our colons contain a lifetime of accumulated waste that our body has not fully released. The colon is also the perfect breeding ground for bacteria and parasites, creating inflammation and toxicity that can negatively affect other organs.

The typical American diet is low in fiber, high in fat, and contains many nonfood items. This diet is dangerous due to the clogging effect these foods have within the colon.

The colon is like a straw or a pipe that runs over 50 percent of the length of your body. Think about what a milkshake does to a straw. A lot of the residuals from the milkshake remain on the inner surfaces of the straw. Just like that straw, the inner walls of the colon over time are lined with lots of residual matter and then baked at 98.6 degrees.

Healthy foods are chemical-free and plant-based.

Exploring the exciting variety of foods available to us from all over the world can easily help us change. The key to a healthy colon is healthy eating. Healthy foods are chemical-free and plant-based. Our diet should consist primarily of fresh fruits, vegetables, and whole grains. Good fats, like olive, fish, and flaxseed oils, are essential. The best sources of protein, carbohydrates, fats, vitamins, and minerals are from plants.

17

A healthy diet is free of fried foods, white sugar, white flour, and excessive meat. These items contain few nutrients and no roughage or fiber to scrub the colon. They also increase the time waste remains within the colon, which increases toxins and the potential for disease.

Meat should be consumed in small portions only a few times a week. Meatless meals are low in fat and cholesterol and can provide all the nutrients needed for a balanced meal. When meat is a part of your meal, be sure to eat an abundance of the quality plant-based foods listed above. These foods help nourish your body and speed up the transit time of the meat through your colon.

> Meat should be consumed in small portions only a few times per week.

Farmers markets, grocery stores, and natural food stores offer a great variety of fruits, vegetables, grains, seafood, and meats.

Fortunately, we now have early detection devices to determine the condition of the colon. As a result, many lives have been saved. However, according to WebMD, a high fiber diet could lower the risk of colon cancer by 40 percent. Eating natural and less processed food is the best way to prevent a health crisis.

------

[*] References:
1. Richard A. Flavell, professor and chair of the Department of Immunology at Yale School of Medicine and a Howard Hughes Medical Institute investigator.
http://medicalxpress.com/news/2011-05-immune-malfunction-trigger-inflammatory-bowel.html.
2. WebMD. *Healthy Eating & Diet*. http://www.webmd.com/diet.

Natural Beauty

What is natural beauty? At one point, it meant still looking great without makeup. It meant not having to work hard at looking good. Beauty and good looks just came naturally. In our fast-paced world today, we seem to have little time to think positively, sleep, eat properly, exercise, or relax. Ironically, these are the secrets to natural beauty.

> The body is the foundation on which we present ourselves. Everything rests upon it.

The cosmetic and beauty industries have exploited this reality with wild promises and products to make you look beautiful again. If you can't grow it naturally, buy it! From nails to breasts, you can buy it. It remains to be seen how much more beautiful we could look if we went back to the basics and used the products and services available to us to enhance the natural beauty that already exists. For example, if you drink eight to ten glasses of water per day and ate more fruits and vegetables, you would have clearer skin. As a result, you would not have to use as much makeup or products that prevent acne or wrinkles.

Begin with the following basic steps and watch what happens to your beautiful look:

Think positively.
Meditate on things that are good. Accepting yourself as a unique designer original is key to a healthy self-esteem and countenance. Don't criticize yourself or others and you will be able to present yourself well. Pray, reflect, and get to

know yourself as a beautiful creation. Self-appreciation is a part of natural beauty. This cannot be purchased.

Take a vacation from the alarm clock.
Sleep several days without the alarm clock. Let your body wake up naturally. To avoid over-stimulating the mind, do not watch TV in bed. Sleep should be a healing time for the body, mind, and spirit.

Eat well for beauty.
Eat more vegetables, fruit, and grains. Drink more water (at least six glasses per day). This flushes the body and helps prevent constipation. Your skin will look better.

Exercise.
Sweat cleanses the body. Exercise tones the muscles and strengthens the frame, which improves posture. Find what works for you and do it at least three times per week.

Relax.
Take a 5- or 10-minute retreat every day to be still. Breathe in and out slowly. As you breathe out, release anything that you need to let go. Once in a relaxed state, your mind will become conscious of what it should let go of or release.

The body is the foundation on which we present ourselves. Everything rests upon it.

Water – To Drink or Not to Drink

Let's face it: plain water has some stiff competition these days. Who wants water when there are sodas, fruit juices, energy drinks, infusions, drinks that are clear, sparkling, smooth, slushy, hot, cold, caffeinated, decaffeinated, with alcohol or without, regular or light? Better yet, who needs water? The answer is: all of us! Drinking water is even more important when we consume these other drinks, most of which dehydrate the body.

> The brain is more than 70 percent water.

The body is more than 60 percent water. But did you know that the brain is more than 70 percent water, the lungs are more than 80 percent water, and blood is 83 percent water? Water is what nourishes and transports oxygen and nutrients to every organ and tissue in the body.

Water also helps produce urine, which is how we eliminate all of the harmful substances that have been extracted from our blood by the filtering process in our kidneys (which are 82 percent water). Although our kidneys will produce urine whether we drink water or not, lack of water requires our kidneys to work much harder.

We can live for about five weeks without protein, carbohydrates, and fats, but only five days without water. Every day, the average adult body loses about three quarts of water. Some nutritionists estimate that 80 percent of Americans are suffering from chronic dehydration.

Ideally, we should get most of our water from eating high-water foods such as raw fruits, vegetables, and their juices. However, most Americans eat mostly concentrated foods that have had the water removed from them by processing or cooking.

An average-size adult should drink at least eight glasses of pure water per day. A good way to determine how much water your body needs is to take your body weight and divide by two. Then drink that amount in ounces of water each day. For example, a five-foot, four-inch woman weighing approximately 130 pounds should consume 65 ounces, or eight 8-ounce glasses, of water each day.

Drinking water at room temperature is best. Cold drinks shock the system. Tap water is a good start. Let the water run for a minute to clear stagnant water sitting in your pipes. If you have concerns about the safety of your water, have it tested by a lab. Spring water is recommended over tap water because it is rich in minerals but low in additives like chlorine and fluoride. Distilled water is the purest form of water and is best during sickness and for internal cleansing.

> If our body is made of mostly water and we never drink water to flush or replenish it, what we end up with is a swamp-like environment in the body.

Even a slight reduction of water in the body can impact our energy level and our ability to think clearly and breathe properly. If our body is made of mostly water and we never drink water to flush or replenish it, what we end up with is a swamp-like environment in the body. No one wants to live near a swamp and no one likes the thought of creating a swamp within his or her own body (dirt, odor, and toxins included).

According to Dr. Fereydoon Batmanghelidj, author of *Your Body's Many Cries for Water,* (Global Health Solutions, 2002), "chronic pains in the body are often indicators of chronic dehydration." It has also been proven that disease of the colon is often caused by dehydration. Dr. Donnica Moore, a specialist in women's health, states that "most people do not know that drinking eight glasses of water daily decreases the risk of colon cancer by 45 percent."

Water helps transport solid wastes and toxins out of the body and aids in the elimination of these wastes through the colon (the large intestine). A diet that consists of fiber, high-water foods (i.e., fruits, vegetables), and water maintains a healthy colon. This diet helps scrape the colon and prevents the clogging that causes disease.

Water is needed for joint and organ health.

The money it costs us every year for doctor visits and prescription drugs is phenomenal. Most of us, at one time or another, have admitted that we do not like drinking water. But think of it as a prescription. Add a slice of lemon. See drinking water as an investment in your body. It is the least expensive and most valuable prescription you will ever buy!

References:
1. Water properties: The water in you. (2015, December 9). Retrieved from http://water.usgs.gov/edu/propertyyou.html.
2. Batmanghelidj F. *Your Body's Many Cries for Water*. Vienna, VA: Global Health Solutions, 2002.

Water and Medication

Many of us take medications every day. The average senior citizen, for example, takes five to ten prescription drugs several times per day.

Unfortunately, many people are not aware that these medications should be taken with a full glass of water. Low body weight, poor diets, chronic dehydration, and taking prescription drugs with just a sip of water could cause major complications, including stomach and urinary problems, headaches, and fatigue.

With the exception of milk (as directed), water—and lots of it—is the only beverage that should be used to take prescription drugs.

The Benefits of Walking

Studies have shown that brisk walking is the best form of exercise for most people because it is already something we do and do well. National health and fitness experts officially embrace the non-strenuous approach to exercise. Other forms of exercise can possibly result in over-exertion, soreness, joint and muscle pain, injury, event planning, and spending money. Walking, on the other hand, is easy, cost effective, and low-impact.

The costs are minimal. A pair of sturdy, supportive shoes and cotton socks are all you need. The perfect shoe should fit so that your arch rests on the shoe's arch. The bottom of the shoe should be rounded to provide a smooth heel-to-toe stride. The shoe should be lightweight and flexible, not so stiff that it prevents the foot from bending naturally.

> We can help prevent and treat disease with regular, moderate exercise.

According to a survey by the Centers for Disease Control and Prevention (CDC) in Atlanta, less than one-third of Americans are active enough for good health. Sixty percent don't exercise regularly and 25 percent don't exercise at all. According to Dr. Harold Elrick, director of the Foundation for Optimal Health and Longevity in Bonita, California, America's seven leading killers are heart disease, cancer, stroke, high blood pressure, chronic obstructive pulmonary disease, diabetes, and osteoporosis. These conditions are responsible for 70 percent of the deaths that occur in the U.S. every year. We can help prevent and treat them with regular, moderate exercise.

Walking 30 minutes a day is adequate, according to the Surgeon General's Report on Physical Activity and Health. It does not have to be 30 consecutive minutes. Small lifestyle changes can help you meet this requirement easily. The CDC and the College of Sports Medicine issued a joint report stating, "If sedentary Americans would adopt a more active lifestyle, there would be enormous benefits to public health and individual well-being." Here are some suggestions:

- Park your car a few blocks farther from your destination and walk the distance.
- Stash a pair of walking shoes in your desk or locker and walk at lunch.
- Become a mall walker (rain or shine).
- Take the stairs instead of the elevator.
- Trade in the power mower for the push model.
- Play tag or hopscotch with your children or grandchildren.
- Start a walking group or get a partner (family member or neighbor).
- Walk your dog.

Regular exercise is essential to good health. It helps you lose weight faster, sleep better, and think more clearly. It boosts your immune system, eases osteoarthritis and back pain, minimizes menstrual and menopausal discomforts, and combats depression and anxiety.

References:
1. Castleman, Michael. *Blended Medicine.* Emmaus, PA: Rodale Book, 2000.
2. Maryland Fitness Council, 2010.

Sleep Hygiene – Healing Sleep

Sleep is essential for a healthy lifestyle. It is the time for cell repair and healing. Sleep is a sacred time. It involves the spirit, mind, and body. We are still, unconscious, and available to the natural order for realignment.

All sleep is not healing sleep, however. Sleep after a heavy meal is not healing sleep because digestion takes priority. Eat three hours before going to bed. If you must eat late, have fresh fruit or a salad instead of fried or processed food. Avoid caffeine and sugar.

Sleep environments must be respected and protected.

The subconscious, which is the seat of our personality, thought, and spirit, never sleeps. For quality rest and sleep, there must be silence—a stillness—that allows the subconscious to be free from distractions. Get your household to agree on the importance of sleep. Turn the telephone off and ask not to be disturbed except for extreme emergencies. When family members are asleep, their sleep environments must be protected until they awaken naturally.

Establish a consistent bedtime. Eight hours of sleep every night is better than 10 hours one day and 6 hours the next. Develop a sleep routine that signals (to the body) that it is time to rest. Avoid reading, eating, or watching TV in bed. It violates your boundaries for sleep vs. daytime activities. Routines like brushing your teeth, bathing, and praying encourage healing sleep.

If falling asleep is difficult, try natural remedies to improve sleep before using sleeping pills. Include an exercise routine. Take a natural calcium supplement for its calming effect, have some chamomile tea before bed, or use other herbs from the natural food store.

Finally, sleep is one of the most important components for healthy living. The effect of sleep deprivation is often underestimated. Healing sleep will add years to your life.

References:
1. Zima Health. Sleep studies statistics.
2. Sleep Disorders Center at the University of Maryland Medical Center. http://www.umm.edu/sleep/sleep_hyg.htm#e.

Health for the Seasons

Seasonal Fasts – Boost Your Immune System

To prepare for the change in season, a juice fast will go a long way. The body needs more energy to adjust to season changes and to maintain a healthy immune system. If we eliminate the digestion of solids, one of the body's largest energy-draining functions, that energy can be reallocated for cleansing, healing, repair, and restoration of other bodily functions.

> The digesting of solids is one of the body's largest energy-draining functions.

A safe juice fast lasts 24 to 48 hours. Use only fresh juices prepared within minutes of consumption. This means you will have to make the juices yourself (you can get a decent juicer for under $80). This ensures that all the nutrients from the fruits or vegetables are available. If juices are heated (pasteurized) or sit on store shelves, most of the enzymes and some of the vitamins and minerals are lost.

Fruit juices are for cleansing the body. The vegetable juices are the builders and restorers of the body. Drink fruit juice in the morning and vegetable juices in the afternoon and evening.

Drink more water. During a fast, the body more rapidly moves stored waste and toxins into the bloodstream for purging. This can cause temporary sluggishness, headaches, and even acne. Drinking more water can help.

Sleep hygiene is also very helpful during a seasonal fast. Eight to 10 hours of restful sleep is recommended.

End your fast with a light meal consisting of fresh fruit, a smoothie, soup, or steamed vegetables.

> Fruit juices cleanse. Vegetable juices build and restore the body.

After fasting, decrease or eliminate consumption of processed foods, alcohol, and tobacco products. A healthy plant-based diet with exercise, proper rest, and healthy thoughts will help the body to detox daily.

Healthy juice recipes can be found at:
http://www.start-living-healthy-recipes-with-tips.com/Juice-Recipes.html

A brief period of less to digest gives the body a break. A seasonal fast is not for weight-loss or religious purposes. It is primarily to detoxify the body and strengthen the immune system. See your health practitioner before fasting.

____

References:
1. WebMD.com
2. Balch, Phyllis A. and James Balch. *Prescription for Nutritional Healing*, 3rd ed. New York: Avery, 2000.

Winter Depression

Many of us have already made a date with seasonal depression. "It happens every year," you might say. Think for a minute on the power of words and the fact that you could say, "Last year I was not ready for winter and it really got me down. This year I am going to prepare myself and not put life on hold just because it is winter!" Wow! How powerful that feels!

> Think on the power of thoughts and words.

Here are some additional liberating thoughts and ideas to help you in your new way of jumping into winter:

Meet winter head-on.
See it coming and plan for it. Embrace it like an evergreen extracting all the freshness and energy of the new season. Don't resist something that is so natural. Flow right into it.

Hibernate.
Understand the purpose of winter and how important it is to your overall health and longevity. It is the time to rest and recharge as much as possible. Go to sleep earlier. In winter your body expects more sleep, which corresponds with nature's longer nights.

Set springtime goals.
Winter won't last forever, so use it as a time to get ready for spring. Out of that goal setting will come many indoor projects leading up to spring accomplishments. These projects could include research, reading, phone calls, inquiries, and planning.

Exercise.
Keep your body loose and fit. Stretch and do some type of exercise that is good for you every day. Open a window and take deep breaths to clear your lungs. The lungs and the large intestine impact health during this season, so keep them clear and mucus free.

Enjoy the "great indoors."
Schedule indoor activities, projects, and free time. Experiment with recipes to make them healthier, and write letters (or e-mails) to catch up with friends and family. Go to the craft shop and pick up that old hobby or start a new one. For example, get out those wonderful vacation or special occasion photographs and scrapbook them. This does several things: it becomes a keepsake, and it will lift you out of your winter blues as you relive happy moments.

Bring nature inside.
To bring cheer to your home, buy freshly cut flowers weekly and place them in a prominent place in the house. Make sure to discard them as soon as they start to wilt. Buy house plants, which provide fresh oxygen and add interest to your interior décor, for several rooms in your home.

Stay positive.
Stop criticizing yourself and others. Add the words, "It's going to be all right" as your everyday affirmation. Find one thing to laugh about every day. Laughter is therapeutic and a great massage for the internal organs.

Limit your screen time.
Don't watch TV before bed or at meals, which is a primary source for reinforcing negative thinking. Buy a few easy listening CDs and get some of that reading done. Schedule TV time—don't let it just trespass over your entire space and time. That gives TV too much power.

Eat foods that beat the blues.
Eat less meat and more fruits, vegetables, whole grains, beans, and nuts. Nature is at rest and living inward. Include

more garlic, onions, beets, ginger, and burdock in your diet. Our bodies respond well to these root foods because of their medicinal properties for building a healthy immune system. Additionally, eat foods that were part of the autumn harvest, such as citrus, apples, grapes, pears, walnuts, sunflower seeds, squash, brown rice, corn, and wheat. Our bodies also respond well to the following spices: turmeric (which is also in curry), fennel, cumin, peppers, sage, nutmeg, and parsley. Limit sweets, cheese, bread, milk, and fried foods, which all promote congestion (mucus) in our bodies.

> Our bodies respond well to root foods during the winter months.

Stay hydrated.
Dehydration is very common during the winter months. Water is an essential nutrient for the brain that promotes positive thinking. Experiment with the wonderful variety of herbal teas, using honey, lemon, or maple syrup as sweeteners if needed. Limit alcohol, which can lead to dehydration. Alcohol weakens body and brain function. Alcohol also makes us more vulnerable to depression.

Take the "winter challenge."
How many layers of clothing will you need in order to stay warm? Keep your chest, neck, head, and feet warm. If winter wins that day, try again tomorrow. Wear a brightly colored item (scarf, hat, or gloves), which is a great pick-me-up for you and others.

Have fun!
Plan at least one winter get-together and invite special people who can bring positive energy into your home.

Notice that these things do not require a lot of money. Meaningful things don't have to break the budget.

If you can implement these suggestions, you can cancel that standing date with seasonal depression. Instead, you will have embraced winter like an evergreen. Winter never felt so good!

―――――
References:
1. Teehee.com. Laugh therapy.
2. Balch, Phyllis A. and James Balch. *Prescription for Nutritional Healing*, 3rd ed. New York: Avery, 2000.

Surviving Holiday Feasts

For many of us, the holiday season brings with it a mixture of issues and challenges. Aside from hits to our budget for glittery outfits and gifts, the next biggest challenge is to avoid overeating and weight gain.

The fact that most Americans suffer from irregular metabolisms makes us more susceptible to weight gain during this time of year. The reason for the season is to appreciate life at the spiritual level, spend time with family and friends, meet people, and do things that we don't have the opportunity to do any other time of the year. Food is used as a common thread and a major element of an affirming, wholesome environment in which to be social.

> Don't be fooled! Most food looks good,
> but not all food is good for you.

Here are a few suggestions that will help you push back from the table and override those impulses to overeat:

Start thinking differently about food.
The holiday season is the perfect time to become a more conscious eater. Conscious eaters don't eat because food is present. They make decisions around food based on what the body needs to be healthy. Appearance and stature are not built solely upon foods that taste good.

Each time you eat, choose a little for taste and a lot for your health and beauty. Don't be fooled! Most food looks good, but not all food is good for you.

Eat colorful foods.
If your meals include fruits and vegetables that are at least three different colors, you have the nutritional properties of a healthy meal. Eat foods that have few ingredients and little processing.

Remember that every non-food ingredient (preservatives, fats, additives, and fillers) that is eaten causes extra work for the body. Prior to digestion, the body must rummage through these non-foods to find nutrients that the body can use for cell development and repair. This extra work takes energy (life) out of the body.

Never arrive to an event hungry.
It is almost impossible to control your food choices when you are hungry. The desire for large volumes of whatever looks and tastes good is too strong. Have a bowl of soup, a piece of fruit, yogurt, or toast. This will send the body a message to stay calm. Use a smaller plate and start with smaller portions. This makes it safer to go back for a little more.

It is almost impossible to control your food choices when you are hungry. Eat a little bit before a large feast to signal to the body to stay calm.

Protect your metabolism.
Many of us skip meals to save calories in an effort to lose weight. Others go on diets that yield rapid weight loss initially (which is probably water loss). These shortcuts put the body into starvation mode, causing an internal crisis and slowing down your body's metabolic rate. Thus, much of what is eaten is stored as body fat.

Trying to lose weight fast is a trap that can destroy your metabolism, which is the manner and rate of speed at which the body uses food. The best way to lose weight is to reduce the overall volume of food eaten at each meal and to eat lots of fresh fruits and vegetables. Animal protein (including dairy) is the major source of cholesterol. Vegetables and grains provide a better source of protein.

Plan your meals.
Develop a food strategy before it is time to eat. Decide what you are going to eat (and drink) and determine your limits before you go out. Remember that the peak energy level for the body is when the sun is most intense (around 11 a.m.–2 p.m.). This is when you should eat your heaviest meal.

If you are eating after 7 p.m., eat less and foods that are lower in fat. If appropriate, prepare a covered dish to contribute to the meal. This ensures that there will be something there for you to eat.

It is no surprise that we will want to eat every four to six hours. Plan your meals in order to avoid food deprivation.

During the holiday season, there is no healthy substitute for self-control and a commitment to eat consciously.

Exercise.
Don't forget to dance! It will ease hunger and increase your thirst. Any kind of dance is a great workout and easy to do during this time of year. A brisk walk or jog (for 15–30 minutes daily) is also good. Regular aerobic exercise is essential for good health and weight control.

During the holiday season, there is no healthy substitute for self-control and a commitment to eat consciously. As time goes on, dieting, improper eating, and poor health can alter your metabolism, making it easy to gain weight.

As you remember the reason for the season, take the high road of self-discipline and make food choices that let you have fun, feel good, and look great the next morning.

The Best Gift You Can Give

The best gift you can give to yourself and to others is a healthy you! All other gifts are symbolic and in no way compare to the time, thought, and presence that comes with you being the best you can be.

A healthy you is a perfect gift you can give to the people you care about and to those who depend on you. This gift is priceless. It extends the time for everyone to benefit from your vibrant energy and zeal. It allows people to learn and experience things that can only come from your unique personality and purpose.

> How you live each day (your lifestyle) impacts the quality of your "health gift."

Each day you live impacts the quality of your "health gift." Daily investments are needed in order to preserve and protect your body from disease and ailments that rob you of quality living. Start now, one day at a time, working on a plan to give the gift of your good health.

To prepare yourself for giving, take an honest assessment of your current lifestyle. For many of us, if we continue our current lifestyles, we will never see our grandchildren. If we do live, we will be remembered as the feeble, sickly ones who had no energy or passion for living.

Here are some things you can do right now to get on the path to a healthier lifestyle:

Nourish your body.
One of the secrets to good health is a plant-based diet. This diet includes fresh vegetables, fruits, whole grains, beans, legumes, and nuts. This type of diet improves digestion and helps the body by giving it the fuel required for proper nourishment and restoration. Meat should make up a very small part of your diet.

Our nation's food supply has been compromised. Mass production and processing have brought more denatured foods to market than ever before. As a result, food supplements like chlorophyll and a multi-vitamin are needed. Also, include essential oils like flaxseed, fish, and olive.

Drink plenty of pure water.
The body is more than 75 percent water and must be properly hydrated every day. Water helps transport oxygen to the cells and is needed to properly eliminate waste. Lack of water can cause headaches, constipation, acne, bladder and kidney problems, and other complications.

If you do not drink six to eight glasses of water each day, set a weekly goal to increase your water intake each day by one additional glass. Each week you should see an improvement in your health. If you are a coffee drinker, know that coffee dehydrates the body. Drink two additional glasses of water for every cup of coffee.

Protect yourself.
Protect yourself from bad food, negative people or things, stress, and toxic substances. The health of your spirit, mind, and body determine your well-being.

Move.
Keep your body fit. Determine what will work for you. What realistically fits into your current schedule without too much disruption? If it is too disruptive to you or your family's routine, it will be impossible to maintain. See your doctor before you start, and avoid injury by starting slowly.

Rest.
Get quality sleep on a daily basis. Sleep deprivation has become a national health issue. Sleep is a major healing component provided for us by the Creator.

Appreciate yourself.
Your good health is your most precious asset. Be your own best friend. As you begin to care for yourself, others will begin to see you in a more positive way as well and value you as the very special person that you are. Remember that we are all born designer originals, but many of us die as imitations of those around us.

We are all born designer originals.

Whatever your state of health is at this time, there are lifestyle changes you can make to help prevent degenerative disease and sickness. A healthier you will not happen instantly. It takes approximately four weeks to develop new habits, so be patient. All changes require sacrifice and planning, but it's worth it.

The best gift you can give is absolutely a healthy you!

Resolutions for a Healthy New Year

When the Christmas tree is down, the Hanukkah menorah is stored, and the Kwanzaa kinara is packed away, we have to come down from the mountain and get back to day-to-day life. This year, however, many of us have come to realize that a healthier lifestyle is essential in order to complete our life's mission and to pursue those things we are most passionate about.

The state of your spirit, mind, and body determines your well-being. The way we care for ourselves and how we allow others to treat us either helps us remain healthy or takes our good health away. We must protect ourselves from bad food, negative people and things, stress, and toxic substances.

> Protect yourself from bad food, negative people, toxic things, and unhealthy activities.

We must stay connected to the source of life, strength, and divine healing. Know that the decision for our existence was decided before time, and that we are living for a very important and specific purpose. The life we live will make an impact for future generations. Once we embrace this larger picture, we will begin to see our true value. Good health is essential for us to complete that predestined work that has been carved out for us to do.

See yourself as a fine tool that must be fit, full of energy, overflowing with peace, contentment, and well-being. This condition cannot survive with a lifestyle of negative thinking, processed foods, little sleep, lots of TV, smoking, and alcohol.

See yourself as a fine tool that must be fit and full of energy.

A healthy lifestyle requires planning and sacrifice. We must remain conscious of our intent to stay healthy every day of the year. We must move gradually but consistently into new routines that turn into habits, which eventually become a part of our personal value system and way of life. Good health is a *lifestyle*, not a passing fad, so let us choose to live life more abundantly in the coming year.

Dealing with Springtime Allergies

For many, spring means allergy season. Allergies are an immune response to a body that is overloaded. Malnutrition and poor health weaken the immune system, making it more susceptible to environmental factors.

The body is constantly exposed to germs on our skin, hands, nails, and hair. Normally, the body can fight them off, but when there is a breakdown in the body's ability to fight off invaders, we begin to feel effects such as sneezing, watery eyes, headaches, and mucus build-up. The problem is an immune system that has been compromised.

> The body is constantly exposed to germs and allergens. Having a strong immune system protects us from these environmental factors.

The body needs quality food in order to heal and repair. The typical American diet, which is low in fiber and high in fat, does not fit the bill. We need chemical-free fruit, vegetables, and whole grains. Also consider the following immune boosters:

- Take two to three teaspoons of locally harvested, unfiltered honey, which contains local pollens. It acts as a vaccine against the pollens that cause allergies. Use in warm herbal tea or lemon water.
- Consider a short one-to-two day fresh juice fast.
- Drink water and fresh fruit juices between meals.
- Exercise and get plenty of rest.
- Take coenzyme Q10 and vitamin C supplements.

- Avoid dairy products before and during allergy season. Use soy or rice milk products.
- Reduce meat consumption.
- Reduce foods made with white flour and refined sugar.
- Do not blow your nose. Prevent sinus irritation by bringing drainage to the back of the throat and expel.

Effective over-the-counter remedies are available at natural food stores. They will support the immune system and eliminate the symptoms altogether. These natural remedies generally have no side effects. Unlike medicines, they leave no residuals (toxins and metals) that accumulate in the body and cause potential problems over time.

Summer Health

During the summer, many of us are exposed to temperatures well over 90 degrees on a consistent basis. Longer days and warm weather revive us in many ways. The warmth of the sun makes our bones and muscles feel better. This is a great opportunity to renew your mind through vacation, retreats, and family gatherings.

> Heat safety is vitally important to our health during the summer months.

To avoid setbacks with your health, here are some things you can do to make moving about in this heat safe and enjoyable.

Be sun smart.
The sun is more intense from 11 a.m. to 2 p.m. Avoid long periods in the sun at that time. If you are taking prescription drugs, know that heavy sun exposure can alter the effects of some medications.

Block the sun.
Wear high-SPF sunscreen with both UVA and UVB blocking power. Not only does sunscreen protect against burns, it helps prevent skin cancer, wrinkles, and age spots. People of color need to wear sunblock, too. The sun's rays also affect eye health, so wear sunglasses with UVA and UVB protection.

Dress appropriately.
Wear a head covering and loose-fitting clothes made of 100 percent natural fibers like cotton, linen, silk, and lightweight

wool. These fabrics allow your skin to breathe, help you stay cooler, and protect you from overexposure to the sun.

Stay hydrated.
Drink plenty of fluids, mostly water. Natural fruit juices help restore the body's vitamin and mineral balance. Coconut water is an excellent hydrating drink. Keep in mind that fluids do not have to be ice cold; room temperature is fine. To avoid dehydration, drink before you get thirsty. Drinks made from sugar or high fructose corn syrup can make you tired and should be avoided.

Avoid overeating.
Instead of three big meals, try eating several small meals consisting of mostly fruits and vegetables, which nourish and cleanse the body.

Enjoy and appreciate every summer day for the gift that it truly is. The energy that comes with warm weather makes us want to become more active. Be active, be careful, and stay healthy.

Staying Healthy in Autumn

Autumn for some of us is that time of year when we are forced to make changes in our daily routine. This can be a challenge for creatures of habit. We often lack the flexibility needed to transition with the seasons.

There are so many visible signs of autumn. Mornings are cooler, days are shorter, and nights are longer. The foliage begins to change and plants and animals are preparing to hibernate.

We are also changing. We may feel that "back to school" pull to get things done and look for the results of what we accomplished over the last few months: our harvest. We begin to look inward and feel a need to plan for the holidays and colder weather. The body is also adjusting; we may crave different food sources and feel more tired.

> **Listen to your body and do what nature is doing.**

To maintain a healthy body and to avoid unnecessary colds and flu, listen to your body and do what nature is doing. Our appetites will increase as the body prepares to hibernate and maintain warmth. It is natural to gain a few (three to five) extra pounds, which serve as a layer for warmth. Always maintain your baseline of fruits and vegetables. Meat eaters will want more meat and dairy. Vegetarians will want more whole grains, nuts, beans, seeds, dairy, and eggs (if used).

Beware of mucus-producing, congestive foods, such as cheese, bread, sweets, and fried food. Include roots and herbs like onions, garlic, ginger, and beets, *Echinacea*, cinnamon, turmeric, fennel, cumin, peppers, sage, nutmeg, and parsley, which help provide your body with a boost of energy.

Activities should include good books, home projects, indoor gatherings, and exercise. The body requires more sleep during cooler months. Limit TV, think positively, and be with positive-thinking people. Remember that the flip side of every negative is a positive. There is good energy and healing with this approach as we embrace the newness of autumn.

Understanding Environmental Health

Conscious living means making choices based on the awareness that our health and the health of the people we love can be affected by our actions. Although many Americans have incorporated healthy eating and exercise into their lives, far fewer of us have taken steps to reduce the number of pollutants and toxins we are exposed to on a daily basis. Although it is impossible to fully control our environments, we can become more aware of the environmental toxins that we can control and take action to consciously avoid them. Doing so is essential for maintaining a healthy immune system and quality living.

> Become more aware of the environmental toxins you can control in your home and work space.

Once we develop an awareness of the harmful effects of environmental pollutants, we begin to consciously make choices based on this information. If there is a risk of being exposed to environmental toxins that we can avoid, we have to ask ourselves, "Is what I am doing worth the negative impact of this exposure? Is there an alternative action I can take that will yield the same results without this exposure?"

Most households have very high toxicity levels caused by flame retardants and chemicals in carpeting, furniture, cleaning products, insecticides, weed killers, garden fertilizers, plastics, air fresheners, synthetic fibers, bath and beauty products, and more. Studies have revealed that there is almost a 50 percent higher chance of a stay-at-home parent getting cancer than those who work outside of the home. We are being poisoned inside our own homes. Consider using white vinegar or baking soda to clean instead of toxic sprays. Use organic lawn and pest control services instead of dangerous chemical-based ones. Kill weeds with table salt and vinegar instead of dangerous chemicals. Try natural essential oils instead of toxic candles and air fresheners. Leave your shoes at the door to avoid bringing in dirt and chemicals like motor oil into your living, healing space.

It is not normal to have many colds per year, a constant runny nose in the winter, or recurring ear infections. These illnesses could be caused by a combination of the food and chemicals (allergens) we are exposed to that push our bodies to their limits. W.A. Shrader, Jr., MD practices environmental medicine, which deals with the consequences of our total interaction with our environments. This includes what we breathe, eat, drink, touch, and even think. "When one has poor health, you can bet the environment has played the major role in causing it," explains Shrader.

> It is not normal to have many colds per year.

Not just one thing that we do compromises our immune system; it is a combination of the things we do and expose ourselves to. Living consciously can help us avoid unnecessary exposure.

References:
1. *Science Daily*. Silent Spring Institute's Household Exposure Study (HES). November 2008.
2. Sante Fe Center for Allergy and Environmental Medicine, Lasted modified April 8, 2006,
http://www.drshrader.com/environmental_medicine.htm.

More books by the author

The Seven Disciplines of Wellness:
The Spiritual Connection to Good Health

Got Cancer? Congratulations!
...now you can start living

For wellness tips and inspiration, visit:

ZimaHealth.com

The7Disciplines.com

StartLivingRecipes.com

Notes